Finding Balance: A Comprehensive Guide to Diets and Weight Loss

In a world where fad diets and quick-fix weight loss solutions abound, it can be challenging to navigate the vast landscape of diets and find an approach that is sustainable, effective, and healthy. The journey to achieving and maintaining a healthy weight requires not only knowledge but also a holistic understanding of our bodies, minds, and overall well-being. It is about finding balance.

Welcome to "Finding Balance: A Comprehensive Guide to Diets and Weight Loss." This book is designed to be your trusted companion on your quest to achieve your weight loss goals in a sensible and balanced way. It aims to provide you with a wealth of information, practical tips, and evidence-based strategies that will empower you to make informed decisions about your diet, embrace a healthy lifestyle, and foster a positive relationship with food.

Rather than promoting any one-size-fits-all approach, "Finding Balance" takes a comprehensive view of diets and weight loss. It recognizes that we are all unique individuals with different needs, preferences, and challenges. It acknowledges that successful weight management is not just about shedding pounds but also about nurturing a healthy mindset, fostering self-care, and adopting sustainable habits for the long term.

Throughout this book, we will delve into various topics related to diets and weight loss. We will explore the science behind different dietary approaches, debunk common myths, and provide practical guidance on creating balanced meal plans and making healthier food choices. We will also address the importance of physical activity, stress management, and sleep in achieving and maintaining a healthy weight.

Moreover, "Finding Balance" goes beyond the mere mechanics of weight loss. It acknowledges the emotional and psychological aspects of our relationship with food and our bodies. It explores strategies for cultivating a positive body image, managing emotional eating, and developing a healthy mindset that promotes self-acceptance and self-care.

The ultimate goal of this book is to empower you with knowledge, tools, and strategies that will help you find your own unique path to balance and well-being. It is not about imposing rigid rules or quick fixes but about equipping you with the resources to make informed decisions and create sustainable lifestyle changes that work for you.

So, whether you are starting your weight loss journey, seeking to break free from a cycle of yo-yo dieting, or simply looking to improve your overall health, "Finding Balance" is here to guide and support you. It is a comprehensive resource that celebrates the diversity of approaches to diets and weight loss, encouraging you to find what works best for your body, lifestyle, and personal goals.

Remember, achieving balance is not a destination; it is a lifelong journey. With the knowledge and guidance provided in this book, you will have the tools and understanding to embark on this journey with confidence and empower yourself to live a healthier, happier, and more balanced life.

Welcome to "Finding Balance: A Comprehensive Guide to Diets and Weight Loss." Let's embark on this transformative journey together.

Introduction

- The challenges of navigating diets and weight loss in a saturated market
- The importance of finding balance and taking a holistic approach to weight management

Chapter 1: Understanding Weight Loss
- The science of weight loss: calories, metabolism, and body composition
- Setting realistic goals and expectations
- The impact of weight on overall health and well-being

Chapter 2: Debunking Diet Myths
- Common misconceptions about diets and weight loss
- Understanding the difference between evidence-based information and trends
- Identifying red flags and misleading claims

Chapter 3: The Fundamentals of Nutrition
- Exploring macronutrients and micronutrients
- Building a healthy plate: portion sizes, food groups, and nutrient balance
- The role of vitamins, minerals, and antioxidants in weight management

Chapter 4: Popular Diet Approaches
- An overview of various diet styles: low-carb, Mediterranean, ketogenic, plant-based, etc.
- Examining the evidence, benefits, and potential drawbacks of each approach
- Tips for selecting a diet that aligns with personal goals and preferences

Chapter 5: Creating Balanced Meal Plans
- Designing well-rounded and nutritious meals
- Incorporating variety, flavors, and cultural preferences into meal planning
- Strategies for meal prepping, grocery shopping, and mindful eating

Chapter 6: Physical Activity and Weight Loss
- The importance of exercise in weight management
- Different types of physical activity and their benefits
- Creating an exercise routine that suits individual needs and preferences

Chapter 7: Managing Emotional Eating
- Understanding the connection between emotions and food
- Strategies for recognizing and addressing emotional eating patterns
- Building a healthy relationship with food and finding alternative coping mechanisms

Chapter 8: Nurturing a Positive Body Image
- Challenging societal standards and embracing body positivity
- Techniques for cultivating self-acceptance and self-love
- Practical tips for improving body image and self-confidence

Chapter 9: Sustainable Lifestyle Habits
- The role of sleep, stress management, and self-care in weight management
- Strategies for developing sustainable habits and routines

- Long-term approaches to weight maintenance and preventing weight regain

Chapter 10: Overcoming Challenges and Staying Motivated
- Strategies for overcoming plateaus, setbacks, and self-sabotage
- The importance of self-reflection, self-compassion, and resilience
- Tips for staying motivated and celebrating milestones along the journey

Chapter 11: Embracing a Balanced Life
- Finding harmony between nutrition, exercise, work, relationships, and personal fulfillment
- The importance of stress reduction, relaxation, and self-care activities
- Developing a holistic approach to overall well-being

Conclusion

- Final reflections on the journey to finding balance
- Encouragement to continue embracing a healthy lifestyle
- Resources for ongoing support and further exploration

The challenges of navigating diets and weight loss in a saturated market

In today's world, it seems like everyone is on a diet or seeking the next miracle weight loss solution. The market is saturated with countless diets, supplements, and programs promising quick and easy results. Navigating this landscape can be incredibly challenging and overwhelming, as it's difficult to discern fact from fiction and determine what is truly effective and sustainable.

One of the biggest challenges is the constant bombardment of conflicting information. Every day, we are exposed to new diet trends and fads that claim to be the ultimate solution for weight loss. From low-carb to high-fat, from fasting to detoxing, it's easy to get lost in the sea of options and wonder which one is right for you.

Another challenge is the pressure to achieve rapid weight loss. Many diets and programs promise quick results, often through restrictive eating or extreme calorie deficits. While these approaches may yield temporary weight loss, they are often not sustainable in the long run and can have negative effects on our physical and mental health.

The marketing tactics used by the weight loss industry further compound the challenge. It's common to see before-and-after photos, celebrity endorsements, and sensational claims that appeal to our desire for a quick fix. These tactics can create unrealistic expectations and lead to disappointment when the promised results don't materialize.

Additionally, there is a lack of individualization in many popular diets. Every person is unique, with different metabolic rates, genetics, and lifestyles. What works for one person may not work for another. Yet, we are often presented with a one-size-fits-all approach that fails to consider our specific needs and preferences.

The saturation of the weight loss market also leads to a sense of information overload. We are bombarded with conflicting advice from so-called experts, influencers, and self-proclaimed gurus. It can be difficult to filter through the noise and find evidence-based information that is rooted in scientific research.

In this saturated market, it's important to approach diets and weight loss with caution and skepticism. It's crucial to prioritize our health and well-being above all else, and to seek sustainable and evidence-based approaches to managing our weight. Consulting with a qualified healthcare professional or registered dietitian can provide valuable guidance and support in navigating the challenges of finding the right diet and weight loss strategy for our individual needs. Ultimately, the key lies in making informed choices, focusing on long-term lifestyle changes, and finding a balanced approach that nourishes both our bodies and minds.

The importance of finding balance and taking a holistic approach to weight management

In our quest to manage our weight, it's important to recognize that it's not just about the numbers on the scale or fitting into a certain clothing size. True health and well-being encompass much more than that. It's about finding balance in our lives and taking a holistic approach to weight management.

Finding balance means embracing a healthy lifestyle that goes beyond just what we eat. It involves nurturing our physical, mental, and emotional well-being. When we focus solely on weight loss without considering these other aspects, we can easily become consumed by numbers and restrictions, leading to a negative relationship with food and our bodies.

Taking a holistic approach means considering all the factors that contribute to our overall health. This includes not only our diet and exercise habits, but also our stress levels, sleep quality, social connections, and self-care practices. All of these factors are interconnected and have a profound impact on our weight and well-being.

Finding balance in our diet means nourishing our bodies with a wide variety of nutrient-dense foods while still allowing ourselves to enjoy the occasional indulgence. It means listening to our bodies' hunger and fullness cues and cultivating a positive relationship with food. It's about finding joy in the process of eating and savoring each bite, rather than obsessing over every calorie or macronutrient.

Taking a holistic approach to exercise means finding activities that we genuinely enjoy and that align with our interests and abilities. It's not about punishing ourselves with intense workouts or pushing our bodies beyond their limits. It's about moving our bodies in ways that feel good, whether that's through dancing, hiking, swimming, or practicing yoga. Regular physical activity not only helps with weight management but also improves our mood, boosts our energy levels, and promotes overall health.

Managing stress and prioritizing self-care are crucial components of a holistic approach to weight management. Chronic stress can wreak havoc on our bodies, leading to imbalances in hormones and cravings for unhealthy foods. Finding healthy ways to manage stress, such as practicing mindfulness, engaging in hobbies, or spending time in nature, can support our overall well-being and help us maintain a healthy weight.

Finally, cultivating a positive mindset and practicing self-compassion are essential. Our thoughts and beliefs about ourselves and our bodies play a significant role in our weight management journey. Embracing self-love and acceptance, and treating ourselves with kindness and compassion, can help us make sustainable and healthy choices.

In conclusion, finding balance and taking a holistic approach to weight management is crucial for our overall health and well-being. It's about nourishing our bodies, nurturing our minds, and caring for our souls. By embracing this approach, we can achieve a healthy weight while also enjoying a fulfilling and balanced life.

The science of weight loss: calories, metabolism, and body composition

Weight loss is a complex process influenced by various factors, including calories, metabolism, and body composition. Understanding the science behind weight loss can help us make informed decisions and adopt effective strategies for reaching our goals.

Calories are units of energy that our bodies use for daily functions and physical activity. When we consume more calories than our bodies need, the excess is stored as fat, leading to weight gain. On the other hand, when we consume fewer calories than we expend, our bodies start using stored fat for energy, resulting in weight loss.

Metabolism refers to the chemical processes that occur in our bodies to convert food into energy. It consists of two components: basal metabolic rate (BMR) and physical activity. BMR represents the energy required to maintain basic bodily functions at rest, such as breathing and organ function. Physical activity, including exercise and daily movement, adds to the overall calorie expenditure. Increasing physical activity can help boost metabolism and aid in weight loss.

Body composition refers to the proportion of fat, muscle, bone, and other tissues in our bodies. It is not solely about weight but rather the distribution of weight. Two individuals with the same weight can have different body compositions based on their fat and muscle percentages. Building lean muscle mass through resistance training can increase metabolism and help with weight loss, as muscle tissue burns more calories at rest compared to fat tissue.

While creating a calorie deficit is key to weight loss, it's important to focus on the quality of the calories we consume. A balanced diet consisting of nutrient-dense foods such as fruits, vegetables, lean proteins, whole grains, and healthy fats provides the necessary nutrients for optimal health and supports weight loss. Additionally, adequate hydration, portion control, and mindful eating practices can contribute to successful weight loss.

It's worth noting that weight loss is a highly individualized process. Factors such as genetics, age, gender, and underlying medical conditions can influence how our bodies respond to diet and exercise. It's important to approach weight loss with a realistic mindset, setting achievable goals and focusing on overall health and well-being rather than solely on the number on the scale.

In conclusion, weight loss involves the principles of calories, metabolism, and body composition. By creating a calorie deficit through a balanced diet and increased physical activity, we can promote weight loss. Understanding these scientific concepts can guide us in making informed choices and adopting sustainable habits for long-term success. Remember, it's important to prioritize overall health and well-being rather than just the number on the scale.

Setting realistic goals and expectations

Setting realistic goals and expectations is crucial when it comes to achieving success in any endeavor, including weight loss or fitness goals. By setting realistic goals, you can avoid disappointment, stay motivated, and make sustainable progress. Here are some tips for setting realistic goals and managing expectations:

1. Assess your current situation: Take an honest look at your current fitness level, lifestyle, and commitments. Consider factors such as your starting weight, fitness level, available time for exercise, and any potential limitations or challenges.

2. Define specific and measurable goals: Rather than setting vague goals like "losing weight" or "getting in shape," make your goals specific and measurable. For example, aim to lose a certain amount of weight or body fat percentage, run a certain distance within a specific time frame, or complete a certain number of workouts per week.

3. Consider your timeline: Set a realistic timeline for achieving your goals. It's important to be patient and understand that sustainable changes take time. Avoid setting overly aggressive timelines that could lead to frustration or unhealthy behaviors.

4. Break it down: Break your larger goal into smaller, manageable milestones. This allows you to track your progress and provides a sense of accomplishment along the way. Celebrate each milestone reached, as it helps to stay motivated and maintain focus.

5. Be flexible and adaptable: Understand that progress may

not always be linear, and there may be setbacks or plateaus along the way. It's important to be flexible and adapt your approach when needed. Embrace the journey and be willing to make adjustments as necessary.

6. Focus on non-scale victories: While weight loss or specific performance goals may be the main focus, don't overlook the other benefits and achievements that come with living a healthier lifestyle. Notice improvements in energy levels, mood, strength, flexibility, and overall well-being. These non-scale victories are just as important and can provide motivation and encouragement.

7. Seek professional guidance: If you're unsure about setting realistic goals or managing expectations, consider seeking guidance from a certified fitness professional, nutritionist, or health coach. They can help you set appropriate goals based on your individual circumstances and provide support and guidance throughout your journey.

Remember, everyone's journey is unique, and what works for one person may not work for another. By setting realistic goals and managing your expectations, you can create a sustainable path towards success and long-term well-being. Focus on progress, not perfection, and embrace the journey towards a healthier and happier you.

The impact of weight on overall health and well-being

The impact of weight on overall health and well-being is significant. Maintaining a healthy weight is crucial for optimal physical, mental, and emotional well-being. Here are some key aspects of how weight can affect our health:

1. Physical health: Excess weight, particularly body fat, can increase the risk of various health conditions, including heart disease, type 2 diabetes, high blood pressure, stroke, certain types of cancer, and musculoskeletal disorders. Carrying extra weight can put stress on the joints, leading to joint pain and mobility issues. It can also impact respiratory function, sleep quality, and overall energy levels.

2. Mental and emotional well-being: Body weight can have a significant impact on mental and emotional well-being. Society's emphasis on thinness and unrealistic body standards can lead to body dissatisfaction, poor self-esteem, and negative body image. This can contribute to the development of eating disorders, anxiety, depression, and other mental health issues.

3. Energy and vitality: Maintaining a healthy weight can improve energy levels and overall vitality. Excess weight can make everyday activities more challenging and exhausting, leading to a sedentary lifestyle and decreased motivation to engage in physical activities. By maintaining a healthy weight, individuals can experience increased energy, improved mood, and a

greater sense of vitality and well-being.

4. Disease prevention and management: Maintaining a healthy weight is an important factor in preventing and managing chronic diseases. Losing excess weight can help reduce the risk of developing conditions such as diabetes, cardiovascular disease, certain types of cancer, and metabolic syndrome. It can also improve the management of existing health conditions and reduce the need for medication.

5. Longevity: Research has shown that maintaining a healthy weight is associated with a longer life expectancy. Excess weight, especially obesity, is linked to an increased risk of premature death. By maintaining a healthy weight, individuals can increase their chances of living a longer and healthier life.

It's important to note that weight is just one aspect of overall health, and individual health is influenced by various factors such as genetics, lifestyle habits, and mental well-being. It's essential to focus on adopting a balanced approach to health, which includes regular physical activity, a nutritious diet, stress management, and self-care practices.

If you have concerns about your weight or overall health, it's always a good idea to consult with a healthcare professional who can provide personalized guidance and support. Remember, small and sustainable changes over time can make a significant difference in achieving and maintaining a healthy weight and overall well-being.

Common misconceptions about diets and weight loss

When it comes to diets and weight loss, there are many misconceptions that can lead to confusion and frustration. Here are some common misconceptions to be aware of:

1. All calories are the same: One common misconception is that all calories are the same, regardless of their source. In reality, the quality of the calories we consume matters. While it's true that calorie intake plays a role in weight loss or gain, the nutritional value of the food we eat is equally important. Nutrient-dense, whole foods provide essential vitamins, minerals, and fiber that support overall health, whereas empty calories from processed foods offer little nutritional value.

2. Fad diets are the answer: Fad diets promise quick and dramatic weight loss results but often fail to deliver sustainable, long-term success. These diets typically involve severe restrictions or elimination of certain food groups, which can be difficult to maintain and may lead to nutrient deficiencies. Additionally, fad diets don't address the underlying factors contributing to weight gain or provide strategies for long-term behavior change. Instead of relying on short-term fixes, it's important to adopt a balanced and sustainable approach to eating.

3. Cutting out entire food groups is necessary: Some diets advocate for the complete elimination of certain food groups, such as carbohydrates or fats. While reducing

consumption of certain types of foods may be beneficial for some individuals, completely eliminating entire food groups can lead to nutrient imbalances and deprive the body of essential nutrients. It's important to focus on moderation, portion control, and choosing nutrient-dense foods from all food groups.

4. Supplements are a magic solution: Many people turn to weight loss supplements or "magic pills" in hopes of quick results. However, these supplements are often not backed by scientific evidence and can have potential side effects. There is no substitute for a balanced diet and regular physical activity when it comes to achieving and maintaining a healthy weight. It's always best to prioritize whole, nutritious foods over supplements.

5. Rapid weight loss is better: Another misconception is that rapid weight loss is better than slow and steady progress. While it's natural to want to see quick results, rapid weight loss can often lead to muscle loss, nutrient deficiencies, and a higher chance of regaining the weight once the diet is discontinued. Sustainable weight loss occurs gradually and involves making long-term lifestyle changes that can be maintained over time.

It's important to approach weight loss and dietary choices with a critical mindset and rely on evidence-based information. Consulting with a registered dietitian or healthcare professional can provide personalized guidance and help separate fact from fiction when it comes to diets and weight loss. Remember, sustainable weight management is about making long-term changes that support overall health and well-being.

Understanding the difference between evidence-based information and trends

In today's world, it can be challenging to navigate through the sea of information and trends surrounding health, wellness, and weight loss. Understanding the difference between evidence-based information and trends is crucial for making informed decisions about your health. Here are some key points to consider:

1. Scientific research and evidence: Evidence-based information is rooted in scientific research and studies. It involves rigorous testing, analysis, and peer-review processes to ensure accuracy and validity. This type of information is based on reliable data and provides a strong foundation for understanding health-related topics.

2. Consistency in findings: Evidence-based information is built upon a body of research with consistent findings over time. Multiple studies and experts in the field will generally support and corroborate the information, providing a level of confidence in its accuracy.

3. Credible sources: When seeking information, it's essential to rely on credible sources such as reputable scientific journals, government health agencies, and registered healthcare professionals. These sources have strict standards and guidelines for publishing information based on scientific evidence.

4. Peer-reviewed publications: Articles that have undergone a peer-review process have been critically evaluated by experts in the field. This process helps

ensure the quality and accuracy of the information presented.

5. Lack of bias and vested interests: Evidence-based information is free from biases or financial interests that may influence the results or recommendations. It is important to consider the source of information and any potential conflicts of interest.

On the other hand, trends are often driven by marketing, personal anecdotes, and popular culture. They may lack scientific evidence or be based on limited research. Trends tend to come and go quickly, often promising quick fixes or drastic results without considering individual differences or long-term sustainability.

To distinguish between evidence-based information and trends, consider the following:

1. Look for scientific support: Assess whether the information is supported by multiple studies, research findings, and expert opinions.
2. Consider the sample size: Studies with larger sample sizes tend to be more reliable as they provide a more representative picture of the population being studied.
3. Evaluate the source: Examine the credentials and expertise of the author or organization sharing the information. Reputable sources will cite their references and sources of information.
4. Beware of red flags: Be cautious of sensational claims, anecdotal evidence, and extreme approaches that promise miraculous results without scientific backing.

Remember, evidence-based information is grounded in research, supported by scientific consensus, and constantly evolving as new findings emerge. By critically evaluating the information you come across and seeking reliable sources, you can make informed decisions about your health and well-being.

Identifying red flags and misleading claims

When it comes to health, wellness, and weight loss, it's essential to be able to identify red flags and misleading claims. Here are some key factors to consider:

1. Quick fixes and miraculous claims: Be wary of claims that promise rapid or effortless weight loss. Sustainable weight loss usually requires long-term changes in diet, physical activity, and lifestyle habits.

2. Extreme or restrictive diets: Diets that eliminate entire food groups, severely restrict calories, or promote excessive and unhealthy behaviors should be approached with caution. A balanced and varied diet is important for overall health and well-being.

3. No scientific evidence or references: Claims that lack supporting scientific studies, references, or reputable sources should raise concerns. Look for evidence-based information that is backed by research and expert consensus.

4. Overemphasis on supplements or products: If a program or product heavily relies on supplements, pills, or other products as the primary solution for weight loss, be skeptical. Weight loss should primarily focus on sustainable lifestyle changes, including diet and physical activity.

5. Personal testimonials as sole evidence: Anecdotal evidence and personal testimonials may not be reliable indicators of effectiveness or safety. Look for a variety of sources and studies to support claims.

6. Unrealistic promises: Be cautious of claims that

guarantee specific weight loss results or claim to target specific body parts for fat loss. Individual responses to weight loss efforts can vary, and there are no shortcuts or magic solutions.

7. Lack of transparency and hidden costs: If a program or product lacks transparency about its methods, ingredients, or costs, it's important to question its credibility. Ensure that you have a clear understanding of what you're getting into and any potential financial obligations.

8. Consultation with healthcare professionals: Seek advice from qualified healthcare professionals, such as registered dietitians or physicians, who can provide evidence-based guidance tailored to your individual needs.

Remember, maintaining a healthy weight and making sustainable lifestyle changes is a long-term commitment. Be cautious of misleading claims, do your research, and seek trusted sources of information to make informed decisions about your health and well-being.

Exploring macronutrients and micronutrients

When it comes to nutrition, understanding macronutrients and micronutrients is essential for maintaining a balanced and healthy diet. Let's explore these two categories of nutrients:

1. Macronutrients:
    - Carbohydrates: Carbohydrates are the body's primary source of energy. They can be found in foods like grains, fruits, vegetables, and legumes. Complex carbohydrates, such as whole grains, are preferred over simple carbohydrates, like refined sugars.
    - Proteins: Proteins are vital for building and repairing tissues, supporting immune function, and producing enzymes and hormones. Good sources of protein include lean meats, poultry, fish, dairy products, legumes, and plant-based sources like tofu and tempeh.
    - Fats: Fats play a role in providing energy, insulating organs, and aiding in the absorption of fat-soluble vitamins. Opt for healthy fats like avocados, nuts, seeds, olive oil, and fatty fish. Limit saturated and trans fats found in processed foods, fried foods, and fatty meats.
2. Micronutrients:
    - Vitamins: Vitamins are essential for various bodily functions, including immune support, bone health, and energy production. They are found in a wide range of foods, such as fruits,

vegetables, whole grains, dairy products, and lean meats.

- Minerals: Minerals are necessary for the proper functioning of enzymes and hormones, maintaining fluid balance, and supporting bone health. Common minerals include calcium, iron, zinc, magnesium, and potassium. Good sources include dairy products, leafy greens, nuts, seeds, and whole grains.

To ensure you're getting a balanced intake of macronutrients and micronutrients:

- Eat a variety of whole foods, including fruits, vegetables, whole grains, lean proteins, and healthy fats.
- Pay attention to portion sizes and aim for balance between the macronutrients in each meal.
- Consider your individual needs, such as age, sex, activity level, and any specific dietary restrictions.
- If necessary, consult with a registered dietitian or healthcare professional for personalized guidance.

Remember, a well-rounded diet that includes a wide variety of foods will help you meet your macronutrient and micronutrient needs for optimal health and well-being.

Building a healthy plate: portion sizes, food groups, and nutrient balance

Building a healthy plate is a practical approach to ensure you're getting a balanced intake of nutrients from different food groups. Here are some tips for creating a nutritious and well-balanced plate:

1. Portion sizes:
    - Aim to fill half of your plate with non-starchy vegetables like leafy greens, broccoli, peppers, or cauliflower. These provide fiber, vitamins, and minerals with fewer calories.
    - Reserve a quarter of your plate for lean protein sources like chicken, fish, tofu, or legumes. Protein helps build and repair tissues and promotes satiety.
    - The remaining quarter of your plate can be dedicated to whole grains or starchy vegetables such as brown rice, quinoa, sweet potatoes, or whole-grain bread. These provide energy and fiber.
    - Remember, portion sizes may vary depending on your age, sex, activity level, and individual needs. Listening to your body's hunger and fullness cues can also guide your portion sizes.
2. Food groups:
    - Vegetables: Include a variety of vegetables in your meals, such as leafy greens, cruciferous vegetables, root vegetables, and colorful

options. They provide essential vitamins, minerals, and dietary fiber.

- Fruits: Incorporate whole fruits or freshly squeezed juices for natural sweetness, fiber, and a range of vitamins and antioxidants.
- Protein: Choose lean sources of protein, such as poultry, fish, lean meats, eggs, legumes, and plant-based options like tofu or tempeh.
- Whole grains: Opt for whole grains like brown rice, quinoa, oats, whole-grain bread, and pasta. These provide fiber, vitamins, and minerals compared to refined grains.
- Dairy or alternatives: Include low-fat dairy products like milk, yogurt, or cheese, or non-dairy alternatives fortified with calcium and vitamin D.
- Healthy fats: Incorporate healthy fats from sources like avocados, nuts, seeds, olive oil, or fatty fish. These provide essential fatty acids and fat-soluble vitamins.

3. Nutrient balance:

- Aim for a variety of foods within each food group to ensure you're getting a wide range of nutrients.
- Consider the colors of your food choices as different colors indicate different nutrient profiles.
- Be mindful of added sugars, sodium, and unhealthy fats in processed and packaged foods. Opt for whole, unprocessed foods whenever possible.

Remember, building a healthy plate is a flexible approach, and it's important to listen to your body's needs and preferences. Consulting with a registered dietitian can provide personalized guidance based on your specific goals and dietary requirements.

The role of vitamins, minerals, and antioxidants in weight management

Vitamins, minerals, and antioxidants play important roles in overall health and can indirectly influence weight management. While they are not direct contributors to weight loss or weight gain, they are essential for maintaining a healthy metabolism and supporting various bodily functions that can impact weight management. Here's how they contribute:

1. Vitamins:

   - B Vitamins: B vitamins, such as B6, B12, and folate, are involved in energy production and metabolism. They help convert food into energy and support the functioning of the nervous system.
   - Vitamin D: Vitamin D plays a role in calcium absorption and bone health. Some studies suggest that adequate vitamin D levels may be associated with healthier body weight.
   - Vitamin C: Vitamin C is an antioxidant that helps protect cells from damage and supports the immune system. It also plays a role in the production of collagen, which is important for healthy skin.
   - Vitamin E: Vitamin E is an antioxidant that helps protect cells from damage. It also supports immune function and may have anti-inflammatory effects.

2. Minerals:

- Calcium: Calcium is important for bone health and muscle function. Adequate calcium intake, along with vitamin D, is crucial for maintaining strong bones.
- Iron: Iron is necessary for the production of red blood cells and oxygen transport. Inadequate iron levels can lead to fatigue and decreased exercise performance.
- Magnesium: Magnesium is involved in over 300 biochemical reactions in the body, including energy production and muscle function. It also helps regulate blood sugar levels and blood pressure.

3. Antioxidants:

- Antioxidants help protect the body's cells from damage caused by free radicals, which are produced as a byproduct of metabolism and exposure to environmental factors. Antioxidants, such as vitamins A, C, and E, as well as minerals like selenium and zinc, are found in a variety of fruits, vegetables, nuts, and seeds.

While vitamins, minerals, and antioxidants are important for overall health, it's important to note that simply increasing your intake of these nutrients will not directly lead to weight loss or weight gain. Weight management involves a combination of factors, including a balanced diet, regular physical activity, and lifestyle habits.

It's best to obtain these nutrients from a varied and balanced diet that includes a wide range of fruits, vegetables, whole grains, lean proteins, and healthy fats. If you have specific concerns or dietary restrictions, consulting with a healthcare professional or registered dietitian can provide personalized guidance on meeting your nutritional needs.

An overview of various diet styles: low-carb, Mediterranean, ketogenic, plant-based, etc.

There are several popular diet styles that people follow for various reasons, including weight management, health benefits, ethical considerations, or personal preferences. Here's an overview of some common diet styles:

1. Low-carb diet:
     - Focuses on reducing the consumption of carbohydrates, particularly refined sugars and grains.
     - Emphasizes foods high in protein and healthy fats, such as meat, fish, eggs, nuts, and avocados.
     - Examples: Atkins, Paleo, and the ketogenic diet.
2. Mediterranean diet:
     - Based on the traditional eating patterns of Mediterranean countries.
     - Includes a high intake of fruits, vegetables, whole grains, legumes, and healthy fats like olive oil and nuts.
     - Moderate consumption of fish, poultry, and dairy products, and limited intake of red meat and sweets.
     - Known for its association with heart health and longevity.
3. Ketogenic diet:
     - A very low-carb, high-fat diet that aims to induce a state of ketosis in the body, where it

burns fat for fuel instead of carbohydrates.

- Requires strict carbohydrate restriction, typically below 50 grams per day.
- Promotes the consumption of foods like meat, fish, eggs, avocados, and healthy oils.
- Commonly used for weight loss and managing certain medical conditions like epilepsy.

4. Plant-based diet:

- Focuses on a primarily plant-based eating pattern, with an emphasis on fruits, vegetables, whole grains, legumes, nuts, and seeds.
- May include limited or no consumption of animal products.
- Can be flexible, with variations like vegetarian (no meat) or vegan (no animal products at all).
- Often chosen for ethical reasons, environmental sustainability, or health benefits.

5. DASH diet (Dietary Approaches to Stop Hypertension):

- Originally designed to lower blood pressure, but also promotes overall health and weight management.
- Emphasizes fruits, vegetables, whole grains, lean proteins (such as poultry, fish, and legumes), low-fat dairy products, and limited saturated fats and added sugars.

It's important to note that individual nutritional needs vary, and what works for one person may not work for another. It's always a good idea to consult with a healthcare professional or registered dietitian before making significant changes to your diet to ensure it aligns with your specific needs, health goals, and any underlying conditions you may have.

Examining the evidence, benefits, and potential drawbacks of each approach

1. Low-carb diet:

    - Evidence: Low-carb diets have been shown to be effective for weight loss and improving blood sugar control in certain individuals, such as those with insulin resistance or type 2 diabetes.
    - Benefits: Can lead to rapid weight loss, reduced appetite, and improved blood sugar control.
    - Drawbacks: May be challenging to sustain in the long term, can restrict certain food groups, and may result in nutrient deficiencies if not properly planned.

2. Mediterranean diet:

    - Evidence: Numerous studies have linked the Mediterranean diet to various health benefits, including reduced risk of heart disease, improved cognitive function, and lower rates of certain cancers.
    - Benefits: Emphasizes whole foods, including fruits, vegetables, whole grains, and healthy fats, which provide essential nutrients and promote overall health.
    - Drawbacks: Requires adherence to a specific eating pattern and may be challenging for individuals who are not accustomed to this style of eating.

3. Ketogenic diet:
   - Evidence: The ketogenic diet has shown promise for weight loss and improving certain health markers, such as blood sugar control and triglyceride levels.
   - Benefits: Can lead to rapid weight loss and reduced hunger due to its high fat and moderate protein content.
   - Drawbacks: Requires strict adherence to very low carbohydrate intake, which can be challenging and may cause nutrient deficiencies if not properly planned. It may not be suitable for everyone, particularly those with certain medical conditions.
4. Plant-based diet:
   - Evidence: Plant-based diets have been associated with numerous health benefits, including lower risk of heart disease, certain cancers, and type 2 diabetes.
   - Benefits: Emphasizes whole, minimally processed foods and higher fiber intake, which can support weight management, overall health, and reduce environmental impact.
   - Drawbacks: It may require careful planning to ensure adequate intake of key nutrients like vitamin B12, iron, and omega-3 fatty acids, especially in strict vegan diets.
5. DASH diet:
   - Evidence: The DASH diet has been shown to lower blood pressure and improve overall cardiovascular health.
   - Benefits: Emphasizes fruits, vegetables, whole grains, and lean proteins, which provide essential nutrients and promote heart health.
   - Drawbacks: May require increased meal planning and preparation, and can be

challenging to adhere to in social settings or when dining out.

It's important to note that the benefits and drawbacks of each approach can vary based on individual needs, preferences, and health conditions. It's advisable to consult with a healthcare professional or registered dietitian to determine which approach is most suitable for you.

Tips for selecting a diet that aligns with personal goals and preferences

1. Identify your goals: Determine what you want to achieve with your diet, whether it's weight loss, improved athletic performance, better overall health, or managing a specific health condition.
2. Consider your preferences: Think about the types of foods you enjoy and the eating patterns that feel sustainable to you. Choose a diet that aligns with your taste preferences and lifestyle.
3. Assess your health needs: Take into account any specific health conditions or dietary restrictions you have. Some diets may be more suitable for certain health conditions, such as the Mediterranean diet for heart health or a low FODMAP diet for irritable bowel syndrome.
4. Seek evidence-based information: Look for diets that are backed by scientific research and have a strong evidence base supporting their effectiveness and safety. Be cautious of diets that make grandiose claims or lack scientific evidence.
5. Consider long-term sustainability: Avoid short-term fad diets that promise rapid results but are difficult to maintain in the long term. Look for a diet that you can see yourself following for an extended period without feeling deprived or restricted.
6. Consult with a professional: If you're unsure about which diet is best for you, it's recommended to consult with a registered dietitian or healthcare professional.

They can provide personalized guidance based on your individual needs and help you make an informed decision.

7. Experiment and adapt: Remember that there is no one-size-fits-all approach to nutrition. It may take some trial and error to find the right diet that works for you. Be open to experimentation and be willing to make adjustments along the way based on your own experiences and feedback from your body.

8. Focus on overall quality: Regardless of the specific diet you choose, prioritize the quality of the food you consume. Opt for whole, minimally processed foods that are nutrient-dense and provide a variety of essential nutrients.

9. Listen to your body: Pay attention to how your body responds to different dietary approaches. Notice how you feel physically and emotionally, and adjust your diet as needed to support your well-being.

10. Remember that flexibility is key: Don't get too caught up in strict adherence to a specific diet. Allow for flexibility and occasional indulgences to maintain a healthy relationship with food and ensure long-term success.

Ultimately, the best diet is one that is sustainable, nourishing, and enjoyable for you as an individual.

Designing well-rounded and nutritious meals

Designing well-rounded and nutritious meals is key to supporting overall health and achieving weight management goals. Here are some tips to help you create balanced and nourishing meals:

1. Include a variety of macronutrients: Each meal should contain a balance of carbohydrates, proteins, and healthy fats. Carbohydrates provide energy, proteins support muscle growth and repair, and healthy fats are essential for various bodily functions.
2. Prioritize fruits and vegetables: Aim to include a colorful array of fruits and vegetables in your meals. They provide essential vitamins, minerals, and antioxidants, while also adding flavor and texture to your dishes.
3. Choose lean proteins: Opt for lean sources of protein such as poultry, fish, legumes, tofu, or low-fat dairy products. These options provide high-quality protein without excessive saturated fat.
4. Incorporate whole grains: Choose whole grain options like brown rice, quinoa, whole wheat bread, and whole grain pasta. These provide more fiber and nutrients compared to refined grains.
5. Include healthy fats: Add sources of healthy fats like avocados, nuts, seeds, olive oil, and fatty fish. These fats support heart health, brain function, and satiety.
6. Don't forget about fiber: Include fiber-rich foods like whole grains, fruits, vegetables, legumes, and nuts. Fiber helps promote healthy digestion, keeps you full for longer, and helps regulate blood sugar levels.
7. Watch portion sizes: Pay attention to portion sizes

to avoid overeating. Use smaller plates, measure ingredients, and be mindful of your hunger and fullness cues.

8. Minimize processed foods: Limit your intake of highly processed foods that are often high in added sugars, unhealthy fats, and sodium. Instead, choose whole, unprocessed foods whenever possible.

9. Hydrate adequately: Stay hydrated by drinking plenty of water throughout the day. Water supports digestion, nutrient absorption, and overall bodily functions.

10. Plan and prepare meals in advance: Planning and prepping your meals ahead of time can help you make healthier choices and save time during busy days. Consider meal prepping on weekends or planning your meals for the week ahead.

Remember, balance and moderation are key. Aim for consistency rather than perfection, and listen to your body's hunger and fullness cues. Consulting with a registered dietitian can also provide personalized guidance based on your specific dietary needs and goals.

Incorporating variety, flavors, and cultural preferences into meal planning

Incorporating variety, flavors, and cultural preferences into meal planning can make your eating experience more enjoyable and sustainable. Here are some tips to help you diversify your meals while honoring your preferences:

1. Explore different cuisines: Experiment with dishes from various cultures to discover new flavors and ingredients. Try recipes from Mediterranean, Asian, Mexican, Middle Eastern, or African cuisines, among others. This can add excitement and diversity to your meals.

2. Incorporate herbs and spices: Herbs and spices not only enhance the taste of your dishes but also offer numerous health benefits. Experiment with different combinations to create unique flavor profiles. Examples include basil, cilantro, cumin, turmeric, ginger, garlic, paprika, and cinnamon.

3. Incorporate a variety of protein sources: There are numerous protein-rich options available that cater to different dietary preferences and cultural traditions. Explore plant-based protein sources like legumes, tofu, tempeh, and seitan, as well as animal-based sources like lean meats, fish, poultry, eggs, and dairy products.

4. Experiment with whole grains: Whole grains are a great way to add variety to your meals while providing fiber and nutrients. Try different grains such as quinoa, bulgur, barley, millet, amaranth, or farro. These can be

used in salads, pilafs, or as a side dish.

5. Embrace seasonal produce: Incorporate seasonal fruits and vegetables into your meals. They are not only fresher and more flavorful but also often more affordable. Visit farmers' markets or consider joining a community-supported agriculture (CSA) program to access local and seasonal produce.

6. Make swaps and modifications: Adapt recipes to fit your preferences and dietary needs. For example, if a recipe calls for a particular meat, consider substituting it with a plant-based protein source or a different type of meat. Experiment with different cooking techniques, ingredients, and flavors to suit your taste.

7. Seek inspiration from cookbooks and online resources: Explore cookbooks and websites that focus on international cuisine. These resources provide a wealth of ideas and recipes to help you incorporate new flavors and cultural elements into your meals.

8. Plan themed meal nights: Set aside certain days of the week for themed meal nights, such as Taco Tuesday, Stir-Fry Friday, or Mediterranean Monday. This approach adds structure and excitement to your meal planning while allowing you to explore different cultural dishes.

9. Get creative with condiments and sauces: Experiment with various condiments, sauces, and dressings to elevate the flavors of your meals. Try making your own homemade versions using different herbs, spices, vinegars, and oils.

10. Keep an open mind and be willing to try new things: Approach meal planning and cooking with a sense of adventure. Be open to trying new ingredients, flavors, and cooking techniques. You might discover new favorites that you never knew you liked.

Remember, the goal is to make meal planning and eating an

enjoyable and sustainable experience. By incorporating variety, flavors, and cultural preferences into your meal planning, you can maintain a diverse and satisfying diet.

Strategies for meal prepping, grocery shopping, and mindful eating

Meal prepping, grocery shopping, and mindful eating are important strategies that can support your overall health and weight management goals. Here are some tips to help you navigate these areas:

Meal Prepping:

1. Plan your meals: Take some time each week to plan your meals and snacks. Consider your schedule, dietary needs, and personal preferences. This will help you stay organized and make healthier choices.
2. Batch cook: Prepare larger quantities of food and portion them into individual servings. This saves time and ensures you have nutritious meals readily available throughout the week. Cook staples like grains, proteins, and roasted vegetables in advance.
3. Use versatile ingredients: Choose ingredients that can be used in multiple dishes. For example, roasted chicken can be used in salads, wraps, or stir-fries. Pre-cooked grains can be the base for salads or served as a side dish.
4. Portion control: Use containers or meal prep containers to portion out your meals and snacks. This helps you maintain portion sizes and prevents overeating.
5. Prep fruits and vegetables: Wash, peel, and chop fruits and vegetables in advance. Store them in containers or bags for quick and easy access. This makes it more likely that you'll reach for them as a healthy snack or for meal

preparation.

Grocery Shopping:

1. Make a shopping list: Create a list before heading to the grocery store to avoid impulse purchases and ensure you have all the necessary ingredients for your planned meals.
2. Shop the perimeter: Most fresh and nutritious foods are found along the perimeter of the grocery store, such as fruits, vegetables, lean proteins, and dairy products. Focus on filling your cart with these items.
3. Read food labels: Pay attention to the nutritional information and ingredient lists on packaged foods. Choose products that are minimally processed and contain fewer additives and preservatives.
4. Buy in bulk: Purchase staple items like grains, nuts, and seeds in bulk. This can save money and reduce packaging waste. Store them in airtight containers to maintain freshness.
5. Stick to your list: Avoid wandering into aisles that contain unhealthy or unnecessary foods. By sticking to your shopping list, you can minimize temptations and make healthier choices.

Mindful Eating:

1. Slow down and savor your meals: Take the time to sit down, relax, and truly enjoy your meals. Chew your food thoroughly and pay attention to the flavors, textures, and sensations.
2. Eat without distractions: Avoid eating in front of screens or when you're engaged in other activities. Focus on your food and the act of eating to better tune into your hunger and fullness cues.
3. Listen to your body: Pay attention to your body's hunger and fullness signals. Eat when you're hungry and

stop when you're comfortably satisfied. Avoid mindless snacking or eating out of boredom.

4. Practice portion control: Use smaller plates and bowls to help control portion sizes. Be mindful of serving sizes and avoid going back for seconds unless you're truly hungry.

5. Enjoy balanced meals: Strive to include a variety of nutrients in each meal. Include lean proteins, whole grains, healthy fats, and a colorful array of fruits and vegetables.

By incorporating these strategies into your routine, you can simplify meal planning and grocery shopping, and foster a healthier relationship with food through mindful eating practices.

The importance of exercise in weight management

Exercise plays a crucial role in weight management and overall health. Here are some key reasons why exercise is important for maintaining a healthy weight:

1. Calorie expenditure: Exercise helps burn calories, which is essential for weight loss or weight maintenance. When you engage in physical activity, your body burns energy, and if you consistently burn more calories than you consume, it can lead to weight loss. Additionally, exercise can help prevent weight regain after weight loss by increasing calorie expenditure.

2. Metabolic boost: Regular exercise can increase your metabolism, which is the rate at which your body burns calories. When you exercise, your body's energy needs increase, and this can help elevate your metabolic rate even after the exercise session is over. Higher metabolic rate means you burn more calories even at rest, which can contribute to weight management.

3. Muscle maintenance: Exercise, particularly resistance or strength training, helps preserve and build lean muscle mass. Muscle tissue is more metabolically active than fat tissue, meaning it burns more calories at rest. By incorporating strength training exercises into your routine, you can help increase your muscle mass, which can boost your metabolism and aid in weight management.

4. Appetite regulation: Exercise can help regulate appetite

by influencing hormones that control hunger and satiety. It can help reduce appetite and cravings for unhealthy foods, making it easier to maintain a healthy diet and manage portion sizes.

5. Improved body composition: Regular exercise can help improve body composition by reducing body fat and increasing lean muscle mass. Even if the scale doesn't show significant weight loss, exercise can lead to positive changes in your body composition, which can enhance your overall appearance and health.

6. Mental and emotional well-being: Exercise has numerous mental and emotional benefits, including reducing stress, improving mood, boosting self-confidence, and promoting better sleep. When you feel good mentally and emotionally, you are more likely to make healthier choices and stick to your weight management goals.

7. Long-term health benefits: Regular exercise is associated with a reduced risk of chronic diseases, such as heart disease, type 2 diabetes, and certain types of cancer. By engaging in regular physical activity, you not only support weight management but also improve your overall health and well-being.

Remember, exercise should be part of a comprehensive weight management plan that includes a balanced diet, portion control, and other lifestyle factors. It's important to find activities you enjoy and make exercise a consistent part of your routine for long-term success in weight management.

Different types of physical activity and their benefits

There are many different types of physical activity, and each has its own unique benefits. Here are some common types of physical activity and the benefits they provide:

1. Cardiovascular or aerobic exercise: This type of exercise gets your heart rate up and improves cardiovascular health. Examples include brisk walking, running, cycling, swimming, and dancing. Benefits of cardiovascular exercise include improved heart and lung function, increased stamina, weight management, reduced risk of chronic diseases (such as heart disease and type 2 diabetes), and improved mood and mental well-being.

2. Strength training: Strength training involves using resistance (such as weights, resistance bands, or bodyweight) to build and strengthen muscles. Benefits of strength training include increased muscle strength and endurance, improved bone density, enhanced metabolism, better body composition, and reduced risk of injuries. It is important for overall physical fitness and can complement other forms of exercise.

3. Flexibility exercises: These exercises focus on improving joint mobility and flexibility. Examples include stretching, yoga, and Pilates. Benefits of flexibility exercises include improved range of motion, reduced muscle stiffness and soreness, enhanced posture, better balance and coordination, and reduced risk of injuries.

4. Balance and stability exercises: These exercises help improve balance, stability, and coordination. Examples include tai chi, yoga, and specific balance exercises. Benefits of balance and stability exercises include reduced risk of falls and injuries, improved posture, enhanced athletic performance, and increased body awareness.

5. High-intensity interval training (HIIT): HIIT involves short bursts of intense exercise followed by brief recovery periods. This type of exercise can be done with various activities, such as running, cycling, or bodyweight exercises. Benefits of HIIT include improved cardiovascular fitness, increased calorie burn, enhanced metabolic rate, and improved endurance.

6. Sports and recreational activities: Engaging in sports or recreational activities, such as basketball, soccer, tennis, hiking, or swimming, provides a combination of cardiovascular exercise, strength training, and skill development. These activities offer both physical and mental benefits, including improved fitness, enhanced coordination and agility, stress relief, social interaction, and enjoyment.

It's important to find a combination of activities that you enjoy and that align with your goals and preferences. Incorporating a variety of physical activities into your routine can help you reap the benefits of different types of exercise and make your workouts more enjoyable and sustainable. Remember to consult with a healthcare professional before starting any new exercise program, especially if you have any underlying health conditions.

Creating an exercise routine that suits individual needs and preferences

Creating an exercise routine that suits your individual needs and preferences is key to staying motivated and consistent with your fitness journey. Here are some steps to help you design an exercise routine tailored to your needs:

1. Set clear goals: Determine what you want to achieve with your exercise routine. Do you want to improve cardiovascular fitness, build strength, lose weight, increase flexibility, or enhance overall well-being? Setting specific goals will help guide your exercise choices.

2. Assess your current fitness level: Evaluate your current fitness level and consider any limitations or health concerns. If you're new to exercise or have any pre-existing medical conditions, it's important to start slowly and consult with a healthcare professional if needed.

3. Choose activities you enjoy: Find physical activities that you genuinely enjoy and look forward to. This could be anything from running, swimming, dancing, cycling, yoga, weightlifting, or team sports. When you enjoy the activities, you're more likely to stick with them long-term.

4. Consider your schedule and availability: Take into account your daily schedule and commitments. Determine how much time you can realistically dedicate to exercise and when it best fits into your routine. Aim

for a mix of shorter and longer workouts throughout the week to keep things varied and manageable.

5. Select a variety of exercises: Incorporate a mix of cardiovascular exercises, strength training, flexibility work, and any other specific activities that align with your goals. This helps ensure a well-rounded routine that targets different aspects of fitness.

6. Gradually increase intensity and duration: Start at a comfortable level and gradually progress the intensity and duration of your workouts. This helps prevent injuries and allows your body to adapt over time. Aim to challenge yourself while still listening to your body's cues.

7. Include rest days: Rest days are as important as exercise days. They give your body time to recover and repair, reducing the risk of overuse injuries and fatigue. Plan regular rest days into your routine to allow your body to rest and rejuvenate.

8. Be flexible and adaptable: Life happens, and there may be times when your routine needs to be adjusted. Be flexible and adaptable, finding alternative activities or adjusting your schedule as needed.

9. Track your progress: Keep a record of your workouts, noting the exercises, duration, intensity, and any other relevant details. Tracking your progress helps you stay accountable and provides motivation as you see improvements over time.

10. Listen to your body: Pay attention to how your body feels during and after exercise. If you experience pain, discomfort, or extreme fatigue, it may be a sign to adjust your routine or seek professional advice.

Remember, the most effective exercise routine is one that you enjoy and can maintain consistently. It's okay to experiment with different activities and routines until you find what works best for you. Be patient with yourself and celebrate your progress along the way.

Understanding the connection between emotions and food

The connection between emotions and food is a complex and multifaceted one. Many people have experienced turning to food for comfort or as a way to cope with stress, sadness, boredom, or other emotions. This relationship between emotions and food can be influenced by various factors, including personal experiences, cultural influences, societal norms, and individual coping mechanisms.

Here are some key points to consider when exploring the connection between emotions and food:

1. Emotional eating: Emotional eating refers to the habit of turning to food in response to emotional triggers, rather than eating for physical hunger. It is often characterized by consuming large quantities of high-calorie, comfort foods. Emotional eating can provide temporary relief or distraction from negative emotions, but it does not address the underlying emotional issues.

2. Triggers and patterns: Emotional eating can be triggered by a wide range of emotions, such as stress, anxiety, sadness, loneliness, or even happiness. It's important to recognize your specific emotional triggers and the patterns or situations that lead to emotional eating. Keeping a food and mood journal can help you identify these patterns.

3. Mindful eating: Developing mindful eating habits can help break the cycle of emotional eating. Mindful eating

involves paying attention to your body's hunger and fullness cues, as well as being present and fully engaged with the eating experience. It involves being aware of your emotions, but also making conscious choices about what and how much you eat.

4. Emotional awareness and coping strategies: Developing emotional awareness is crucial for understanding and managing the connection between emotions and food. It involves recognizing and acknowledging your emotions without judgment. Finding alternative coping strategies for dealing with emotions, such as engaging in physical activity, practicing relaxation techniques, seeking support from loved ones, or pursuing hobbies, can be helpful in reducing reliance on food as a coping mechanism.

5. Building a healthy relationship with food: It's important to cultivate a balanced and nourishing relationship with food. This involves recognizing that food is not just about physical nourishment but also plays a role in social connections, cultural traditions, and personal enjoyment. Adopting a flexible approach to eating, including incorporating a variety of nutritious foods and allowing for occasional treats, can support a positive relationship with food.

6. Seeking support: If you find that emotional eating is significantly impacting your well-being or if you're struggling to manage your emotions, it may be helpful to seek support from a therapist, counselor, or registered dietitian. They can provide guidance, tools, and strategies to help you develop healthier coping mechanisms and a more balanced relationship with food.

Remember, everyone's relationship with food and emotions is unique. It's important to approach this topic with compassion and self-acceptance. Be patient with yourself as you navigate the complex interplay between emotions and food, and seek the support you need to cultivate a healthier and more balanced approach to eating and emotional well-being.

<h1 style="text-align:center; font-style:italic;">Strategies for recognizing and addressing emotional eating patterns</h1>

Recognizing and addressing emotional eating patterns can be an important step in developing a healthier relationship with food. Here are some strategies to help you become more aware of emotional eating patterns and address them:

1. Identify triggers: Pay attention to the situations, events, or emotions that often lead to emotional eating. Keep a food and mood journal to track your eating habits and the emotions you experience before, during, and after eating. Look for patterns and common triggers that may be linked to emotional eating.

2. Practice mindful eating: Mindful eating involves paying attention to your body's hunger and fullness cues, as well as your emotions and thoughts while eating. Slow down and savor each bite, and take the time to notice the taste, texture, and satisfaction of the food. Mindful eating can help you become more aware of your eating patterns and emotions.

3. Find alternative coping strategies: Instead of turning to food when you're experiencing strong emotions, try finding other ways to cope. Engage in activities that you enjoy and that help you relax or relieve stress, such as exercising, practicing deep breathing, journaling, taking a walk, or talking to a friend. Experiment with different strategies and find what works best for you.

4. Practice self-care: Taking care of yourself in non-food-related ways can help reduce emotional eating. Make

sure you're getting enough sleep, managing stress, and engaging in activities that bring you joy and fulfillment. Prioritize self-care practices that support your overall well-being.

5. Challenge negative thoughts: Negative thoughts or beliefs about food, body image, or emotions can contribute to emotional eating. Practice challenging and reframing these thoughts. Replace negative self-talk with positive affirmations and remind yourself that food does not define your worth or value as a person.

6. Seek support: If emotional eating is a significant challenge for you, consider seeking support from a therapist, counselor, or registered dietitian. They can provide guidance, tools, and strategies tailored to your specific needs and help you address the underlying emotional issues driving your eating patterns.

7. Build a balanced relationship with food: Strive to develop a healthy and balanced approach to eating. Focus on nourishing your body with a variety of nutritious foods while allowing yourself to enjoy occasional treats. Avoid labeling foods as "good" or "bad," and practice moderation and portion control.

Remember, addressing emotional eating takes time and practice. Be patient and compassionate with yourself as you work through these patterns. Celebrate small victories along the way and remember that you are taking important steps toward developing a healthier relationship with food and your emotions.

Building a healthy relationship with food and finding alternative coping mechanisms

Building a healthy relationship with food and finding alternative coping mechanisms can help you break free from emotional eating patterns. Here are some strategies to consider:

1. Practice intuitive eating: Instead of following strict diets or rigid food rules, practice listening to your body's hunger and fullness cues. Eat when you're physically hungry and stop when you're comfortably satisfied. Pay attention to how different foods make you feel and honor your cravings in moderation.

2. Focus on nourishment: Shift your mindset from viewing food as a source of comfort or stress relief to seeing it as fuel for your body. Prioritize nutrient-dense foods that provide the energy and nutrients your body needs to function at its best. Include a balance of fruits, vegetables, whole grains, lean proteins, and healthy fats in your meals.

3. Develop healthy coping mechanisms: Instead of turning to food when you're stressed, anxious, or bored, find alternative coping mechanisms that support your well-being. Engage in activities that help you relax, such as practicing deep breathing, meditation, yoga, or engaging in hobbies that bring you joy. Find healthy ways to manage emotions, such as talking to a friend or therapist, journaling, or engaging in physical activity.

4. Build a support network: Surround yourself with people who support your journey to a healthy relationship

with food. Share your struggles and successes with trusted friends or family members, or consider joining a support group or seeking guidance from a registered dietitian or therapist who specializes in disordered eating or emotional eating.

5. Practice self-care: Taking care of your overall well-being can help reduce the urge to turn to food for comfort. Prioritize self-care activities that help you relax, de-stress, and recharge. This may include getting enough sleep, engaging in regular exercise, spending time in nature, practicing mindfulness, or pursuing hobbies and activities that bring you joy.

6. Challenge distorted thoughts: Pay attention to negative or distorted thoughts you may have about food, body image, or emotions. Practice challenging and reframing these thoughts. Remind yourself that your worth is not determined by your appearance or what you eat. Replace negative self-talk with positive affirmations and focus on cultivating self-acceptance and self-compassion.

7. Seek professional help if needed: If emotional eating continues to be a challenge despite your best efforts, consider seeking support from a registered dietitian, therapist, or counselor who specializes in emotional eating. They can help you explore the underlying emotional triggers and provide strategies tailored to your specific needs.

Remember, building a healthy relationship with food takes time and effort. Be patient with yourself and celebrate small victories along the way. Embrace the journey of discovering alternative coping mechanisms that nourish your body and support your overall well-being.

Challenging societal standards and embracing body positivity

Challenging societal standards and embracing body positivity is an important aspect of developing a healthy relationship with food and body image. Here are some strategies for doing so:

1. Recognize the influence of media: Be aware of how media and societal messages shape our perceptions of beauty and body ideals. Understand that these standards are often unrealistic and unattainable for most people. Limit your exposure to media that promotes unrealistic body standards and seek out diverse representations of beauty.
2. Shift your focus to health and well-being: Instead of obsessing over weight or appearance, prioritize your overall health and well-being. Focus on nourishing your body with balanced meals, engaging in regular physical activity that you enjoy, and practicing self-care. Remember that health looks different for every individual and cannot be determined solely by size or weight.
3. Surround yourself with positive influences: Surround yourself with people who support body positivity and reject harmful diet culture. Seek out communities, online or offline, that celebrate diverse bodies and promote self-acceptance. Engage in conversations that challenge harmful beauty standards and promote body inclusivity.
4. Practice self-acceptance and self-compassion: Embrace

and celebrate your body as it is right now. Shift your mindset from self-criticism to self-acceptance and self-love. Practice positive affirmations, gratitude, and mindfulness to cultivate a more compassionate and accepting attitude toward your body.

5. Engage in positive body image activities: Seek out activities that promote body acceptance and appreciation. This may include engaging in body-positive workouts, participating in body-positive events or campaigns, or following social media accounts that promote body diversity and body positivity.

6. Challenge negative self-talk: Pay attention to the way you talk to yourself about your body. Replace negative self-talk with positive affirmations and practice reframing negative thoughts. Focus on your body's strengths, abilities, and the things it allows you to do, rather than its appearance.

7. Educate yourself on body positivity and related topics: Learn more about body positivity, fat acceptance, and related movements. Read books, listen to podcasts, and follow social media accounts that promote body acceptance and challenge societal beauty standards. Educating yourself can help you gain a deeper understanding and perspective on these topics.

Remember that embracing body positivity is a journey, and it may take time to undo the influence of societal standards. Be patient and kind to yourself as you work towards accepting and loving your body just as it is. Focus on self-care, self-acceptance, and surrounding yourself with positive influences that celebrate and support body diversity.

Techniques for cultivating self-acceptance and self-love

Cultivating self-acceptance and self-love is a lifelong journey that involves practicing self-care, developing a positive mindset, and embracing your true self. Here are some techniques that can help in this process:

1. Practice self-compassion: Treat yourself with the same kindness and understanding you would extend to a loved one. Acknowledge and accept your flaws and imperfections without judgment. Remind yourself that it's okay to make mistakes and that you are deserving of love and understanding.

2. Challenge negative self-talk: Become aware of your negative self-talk and work on replacing it with positive and empowering thoughts. Catch yourself when you start to criticize or belittle yourself and consciously choose to reframe those thoughts in a more compassionate and supportive way.

3. Celebrate your strengths and accomplishments: Focus on your strengths, talents, and accomplishments. Celebrate your successes, no matter how big or small they may be. Recognize the unique qualities that make you who you are and appreciate them.

4. Practice gratitude: Cultivate a mindset of gratitude by regularly acknowledging and expressing gratitude for the positive aspects of your life. Take time to appreciate your body, your health, your relationships, and the opportunities you have been given.

5. Engage in self-care activities: Prioritize self-care and make time for activities that nourish your mind, body, and soul. This can include things like taking walks in nature, practicing mindfulness or meditation, journaling, engaging in hobbies you enjoy, or pampering yourself with a relaxing bath or self-care routine.

6. Set boundaries: Establish healthy boundaries in your relationships and learn to say no to things that don't serve your well-being. By setting boundaries, you prioritize your own needs and create a space for self-acceptance and self-care.

7. Surround yourself with positive influences: Surround yourself with people who uplift and support you. Seek out relationships and communities that promote self-acceptance and positivity. Engage with social media accounts, books, and other media that inspire and encourage self-love.

8. Practice self-care rituals: Develop self-care rituals that make you feel good and promote self-acceptance. This could include daily affirmations, engaging in creative activities, practicing self-compassion exercises, or participating in activities that bring you joy and fulfillment.

9. Embrace self-expression: Find ways to express yourself authentically and embrace your unique qualities. Explore your passions, engage in creative outlets, and express yourself through art, music, writing, or any other form of self-expression that resonates with you.

10. Seek support when needed: Don't hesitate to seek support from trusted friends, family members, or professionals if you're struggling with self-acceptance or self-love. Therapy or counseling can provide valuable guidance and tools for building a stronger sense of self and cultivating self-acceptance.

Remember that self-acceptance and self-love are ongoing

practices, and it's normal to have ups and downs along the way. Be patient and gentle with yourself, and remember that you are worthy of love and acceptance just as you are.

Practical tips for improving body image and self-confidence

Improving body image and self-confidence is a personal and ongoing journey. Here are some practical tips that can help:

1. Practice self-care: Take care of your physical, mental, and emotional well-being. Engage in activities that make you feel good and prioritize your self-care needs.

2. Surround yourself with positivity: Surround yourself with people who uplift and support you. Seek out relationships and communities that promote body positivity and self-acceptance.

3. Challenge societal beauty standards: Recognize that beauty comes in all shapes, sizes, and forms. Challenge societal beauty standards by celebrating diversity and embracing different body types.

4. Focus on what your body can do: Shift your focus from appearance to functionality. Appreciate and celebrate what your body is capable of doing, whether it's through physical activities, hobbies, or daily tasks.

5. Practice gratitude for your body: Cultivate a mindset of gratitude for your body. Focus on the things you appreciate about your body, such as its strength, resilience, and the experiences it allows you to have.

6. Limit exposure to negative media: Be mindful of the media you consume and how it influences your body image. Limit exposure to media that promotes unrealistic beauty ideals or makes you feel inadequate.

7. Practice positive self-talk: Replace negative self-talk

with positive and affirming statements. Be kind and compassionate toward yourself and challenge negative thoughts or criticisms.

8. Engage in body-positive activities: Seek out body-positive activities that help you appreciate and connect with your body. This could include yoga, dance, mindful movement, or any form of exercise that feels empowering and enjoyable.

9. Dress in a way that makes you feel confident: Wear clothes that make you feel comfortable and confident in your own skin. Dress in a way that reflects your personal style and expresses your uniqueness.

10. Seek support when needed: If negative body image or low self-confidence persist, consider seeking support from a therapist or counselor who specializes in body image and self-esteem. They can provide guidance and tools to help you navigate and improve your body image.

Remember that building body confidence takes time and effort. Be patient with yourself and practice self-compassion along the way. Celebrate your uniqueness and focus on your inner qualities and strengths, as they contribute to your overall self-confidence and well-being.

The role of sleep, stress management, and self-care in weight management

Sleep, stress management, and self-care play crucial roles in weight management. Here's a breakdown of their significance:

1. Sleep: Quality sleep is essential for overall health and weight management. Lack of sleep can disrupt hormonal balance, leading to increased appetite and cravings, decreased satiety, and reduced energy expenditure. Aim for 7-9 hours of quality sleep each night to support healthy weight management.

2. Stress management: Chronic stress can contribute to weight gain and hinder weight loss efforts. When stressed, the body releases cortisol, a hormone that can increase appetite, promote fat storage, and affect food choices. Engage in stress-reducing activities such as exercise, mindfulness, meditation, deep breathing, and hobbies to manage stress levels effectively.

3. Self-care: Prioritizing self-care is vital for maintaining a healthy lifestyle and managing weight. Engaging in activities that promote relaxation, pleasure, and emotional well-being can help reduce emotional eating, improve body image, and enhance overall satisfaction. Examples include taking leisurely walks, enjoying a hot bath, reading a book, practicing mindfulness, or spending time with loved ones.

By prioritizing quality sleep, implementing effective stress management techniques, and practicing regular self-care, individuals can better regulate their hormones, reduce emotional eating, make healthier food choices, and manage weight more effectively. Remember that each person's needs and strategies for sleep, stress management, and self-care may vary, so it's important to find what works best for you and incorporate these practices into your daily routine.

Strategies for developing sustainable habits and routines

Developing sustainable habits and routines is crucial for long-term weight management. Here are some strategies to help you establish sustainable practices:

1. Start small: Begin by implementing small changes rather than trying to overhaul your entire lifestyle all at once. Focus on one or two habits at a time, such as drinking more water or adding more vegetables to your meals, and gradually build from there.

2. Set realistic and achievable goals: Make sure your goals are attainable and measurable. Setting realistic targets helps you stay motivated and prevents feelings of discouragement. Break larger goals into smaller, manageable steps to make them more achievable.

3. Create a routine: Establishing a consistent routine can help you maintain healthy habits. Plan your meals, schedule regular exercise sessions, and set aside time for self-care and stress management activities. Consistency will make it easier to stick to your plan and develop sustainable habits over time.

4. Prioritize balance and moderation: Avoid extreme diets or restrictive eating patterns that are difficult to maintain in the long run. Instead, focus on incorporating a variety of nutritious foods into your diet and allowing yourself occasional treats in moderation. Strive for balance and a flexible approach to eating that can be sustained over time.

5. Practice mindful eating: Pay attention to your body's hunger and fullness cues, and eat slowly and mindfully. This helps you develop a better connection with your body and recognize when you're satisfied, preventing overeating or emotional eating.
6. Find enjoyment in physical activity: Choose activities that you genuinely enjoy to make exercise a sustainable part of your routine. Try different forms of exercise until you find something that you look forward to and find fulfilling. This will make it easier to stick to your exercise routine and maintain an active lifestyle.
7. Seek support and accountability: Engage with a supportive community or enlist the help of a friend, family member, or a professional, such as a registered dietitian or personal trainer, who can provide guidance and keep you accountable. Having a support system can provide motivation, encouragement, and help you stay on track with your goals.

Remember, sustainable habits take time to develop, and it's normal to experience setbacks along the way. Be patient with yourself, celebrate your progress, and keep adjusting your routines as needed. By focusing on long-term sustainable habits, you can achieve and maintain a healthy weight and overall well-being.

Long-term approaches to weight maintenance and preventing weight regain

Long-term weight maintenance and preventing weight regain require a comprehensive approach that goes beyond just focusing on diet and exercise. Here are some strategies to help you maintain your weight loss and prevent regain over the long term:

1. Establish realistic and sustainable habits: Focus on developing healthy habits that you can maintain for the long haul. Avoid restrictive diets or extreme exercise routines that are difficult to sustain. Instead, find a balanced approach that includes a variety of nutritious foods and enjoyable physical activities.

2. Monitor your progress: Regularly track your weight, body measurements, and other relevant indicators of progress to stay aware of any changes. This can help you catch any upward trends early on and make necessary adjustments to your habits.

3. Stay active: Regular physical activity is essential for weight maintenance. Find activities that you enjoy and that fit into your lifestyle. Aim for a combination of cardiovascular exercise, strength training, and flexibility exercises. Consistency is key, so make exercise a regular part of your routine.

4. Practice portion control: Be mindful of portion sizes to avoid overeating. Use smaller plates and bowls, and listen to your body's hunger and fullness cues. Practice mindful eating by eating slowly, savoring each bite, and paying attention to your body's signals of satisfaction.

5. Maintain a balanced diet: Focus on consuming a variety of nutrient-dense foods, including fruits, vegetables, whole grains, lean proteins, and healthy fats. Aim for a balanced distribution of macronutrients (carbohydrates, proteins, and fats) to support your overall health and weight maintenance.

6. Manage stress: Chronic stress can contribute to weight regain. Find healthy ways to manage stress, such as practicing relaxation techniques, engaging in hobbies, spending time in nature, or seeking support from friends, family, or a therapist.

7. Prioritize sleep: Aim for adequate sleep each night, as poor sleep can disrupt your appetite-regulating hormones and lead to weight gain. Establish a regular sleep routine, create a conducive sleep environment, and practice good sleep hygiene habits.

8. Seek support: Surround yourself with a supportive network of friends, family, or a support group who can provide encouragement, accountability, and understanding. Consider working with a registered dietitian or a weight management specialist who can provide guidance tailored to your specific needs.

9. Practice self-care: Take care of your mental and emotional well-being. Engage in activities that bring you joy, practice self-compassion, and prioritize self-care. This can help prevent emotional eating and promote overall well-being.

10. Stay flexible and adapt: Recognize that your weight may fluctuate naturally over time. Be flexible and willing to adjust your habits as needed. Life circumstances, such as changes in work, family, or health, may require adaptations to your routine. Embrace these changes and find strategies that work for you.

Remember, weight maintenance is an ongoing journey that requires patience, self-compassion, and commitment. Focus on sustainable habits, prioritize your overall well-being, and embrace a long-term perspective to help prevent weight regain and live a healthy, balanced life.

Strategies for overcoming plateaus, setbacks, and self-sabotage

Plateaus, setbacks, and self-sabotage are common challenges on the weight management journey. Here are some strategies to help you overcome these obstacles and stay on track:

1. Reassess your goals: Take a moment to reflect on your goals and make sure they are still aligned with your values and motivations. If necessary, adjust your goals to make them more realistic or meaningful.
2. Mix up your routine: Plateaus can occur when your body adapts to your current exercise and diet regimen. Shake things up by trying new activities, changing your exercise intensity or duration, or experimenting with different healthy foods and recipes.
3. Stay consistent: Consistency is key to overcoming plateaus and setbacks. Stick to your healthy habits even when progress feels slow or when setbacks occur. Remember that small, consistent efforts can add up over time.
4. Keep a food and exercise journal: Tracking your food intake and exercise can provide valuable insights into your habits and help you identify patterns or areas for improvement. It can also help you stay accountable to your goals.
5. Seek support: Reach out to a friend, family member, or a support group for encouragement and accountability. Having someone to share your challenges and successes with can make a big difference in staying motivated and

overcoming setbacks.

6. Reframe setbacks as learning opportunities: Instead of viewing setbacks as failures, see them as opportunities for growth and learning. Identify what went wrong, analyze the triggers or obstacles, and develop strategies to prevent similar setbacks in the future.

7. Practice self-compassion: Be kind to yourself during plateaus or setbacks. Remember that everyone experiences ups and downs on their journey. Treat yourself with compassion, forgiveness, and understanding. Focus on the progress you have made rather than dwelling on setbacks.

8. Identify and address self-sabotaging behaviors: Be aware of any self-sabotaging behaviors or thought patterns that may be hindering your progress. This could include emotional eating, negative self-talk, or self-sabotaging beliefs. Work on developing healthier coping mechanisms and challenging negative thoughts.

9. Celebrate non-scale victories: Don't solely rely on the scale to measure your progress. Celebrate non-scale victories such as increased energy, improved strength, better sleep, or positive changes in body composition. Recognize and appreciate the positive changes you are experiencing beyond just the number on the scale.

10. Stay motivated with rewards and incentives: Set small, achievable milestones along your journey and reward yourself when you reach them. This can help boost motivation and give you something to look forward to. Choose rewards that are aligned with your health and fitness goals, such as a new workout outfit or a relaxing self-care activity.

Remember that overcoming plateaus, setbacks, and self-sabotage is part of the process. Stay committed, be patient with yourself, and embrace the journey. With perseverance and a positive mindset, you can navigate through these challenges and continue making progress towards your goals.

The importance of self-reflection, self-compassion, and resilience

Self-reflection, self-compassion, and resilience are essential elements for a healthy and sustainable approach to weight management. Here's why they are important:

1. Self-reflection: Self-reflection involves taking the time to examine your thoughts, feelings, and behaviors related to your weight management journey. It allows you to gain insight into your motivations, triggers, and patterns. By understanding yourself better, you can make more informed choices and identify areas for growth and improvement.

2. Self-compassion: Self-compassion involves treating yourself with kindness, understanding, and acceptance, especially during challenging times. It means acknowledging that setbacks and imperfections are part of being human and extending the same kindness and compassion to yourself that you would to a friend. Self-compassion allows you to approach weight management from a place of self-care and non-judgment, which promotes a healthier relationship with food, exercise, and your body.

3. Resilience: Resilience is the ability to bounce back from setbacks, adapt to changes, and persevere in the face of challenges. In weight management, setbacks and plateaus are common, and it's important to develop resilience to keep going. Resilience allows you to learn from setbacks, adjust your approach, and

stay committed to your goals, even when faced with obstacles. It helps you maintain a positive mindset and prevents discouragement or giving up.

By incorporating self-reflection, self-compassion, and resilience into your weight management journey, you can cultivate a healthier mindset, increase your motivation, and navigate challenges more effectively. Here are some strategies to help you develop these qualities:

- Practice mindfulness: Engage in activities such as meditation, deep breathing exercises, or journaling to cultivate self-awareness and become more attuned to your thoughts, emotions, and behaviors.
- Cultivate self-compassion: Treat yourself with kindness, speak to yourself in a supportive manner, and practice self-care activities that promote emotional well-being.
- Set realistic expectations: Avoid setting overly rigid or perfectionistic goals. Instead, set realistic and achievable milestones that allow for flexibility and adaptability.
- Focus on strengths and progress: Celebrate your successes, no matter how small, and recognize the progress you've made. Acknowledge your efforts and improvements rather than dwelling on setbacks or perceived failures.
- Seek support: Surround yourself with a support network of friends, family, or a weight management group who can provide encouragement, accountability, and understanding.
- Learn from setbacks: Instead of viewing setbacks as failures, view them as opportunities for growth and learning. Identify what you can learn from the experience and how you can adjust your approach moving forward.
- Practice self-care: Engage in activities that nourish your

mind, body, and soul. This may include activities like getting enough sleep, engaging in hobbies, spending time with loved ones, or engaging in relaxation techniques.

Remember, weight management is a journey, and it's important to be kind to yourself along the way. Self-reflection, self-compassion, and resilience will help you navigate the challenges, stay motivated, and maintain a positive and balanced approach to your overall well-being.

Tips for staying motivated and celebrating milestones along the journey

Staying motivated and celebrating milestones are essential for maintaining a positive mindset and long-term success in your weight management journey. Here are some tips to help you stay motivated and celebrate your accomplishments along the way:

1. Set specific and achievable goals: Break down your weight management journey into smaller, achievable goals. Set both short-term and long-term goals that are specific, measurable, attainable, relevant, and time-bound (SMART). This will give you a clear sense of direction and something to strive for.
2. Track your progress: Keep a record of your progress, whether it's tracking your weight, measurements, or other relevant data. This will allow you to see your progress over time and provide a visual reminder of how far you've come.
3. Celebrate milestones: When you reach a milestone, take the time to celebrate and acknowledge your achievement. It could be treating yourself to a non-food reward, such as buying new workout clothes, getting a massage, or going on a weekend getaway. Celebrating milestones reinforces positive behavior and provides a sense of accomplishment.
4. Find your motivation: Identify what motivates you personally and use it as fuel to keep going. It could be improving your overall health, feeling more confident in your body, participating in a specific event or activity, or

setting a positive example for your loved ones. Remind yourself of your motivation regularly to stay focused and committed.

5. Surround yourself with support: Seek support from friends, family, or a weight management group who can cheer you on, offer encouragement, and provide accountability. Share your goals and milestones with them, and let them be a source of motivation and celebration.

6. Create a positive environment: Surround yourself with positive influences that align with your goals. This could include following social media accounts that promote a healthy lifestyle, joining online communities focused on weight management, or surrounding yourself with friends who support your journey.

7. Find enjoyment in the process: Engage in activities that you enjoy and that make you feel good. Whether it's trying new recipes, exploring different types of physical activity, or finding ways to incorporate movement into your daily routine, finding joy in the process will help you stay motivated and make the journey more enjoyable.

8. Practice self-care: Take care of yourself holistically by prioritizing self-care activities that promote physical, mental, and emotional well-being. This could include getting enough sleep, managing stress, practicing relaxation techniques, and engaging in activities that bring you joy and rejuvenation.

Remember that motivation may ebb and flow throughout your journey. On days when motivation is low, remind yourself of your goals, reflect on the progress you've made, and use strategies like visualization or positive self-talk to reignite your motivation. Celebrate your milestones, no matter how small, as each step forward is an achievement worth acknowledging.

Finding harmony between nutrition, exercise, work, relationships, and personal fulfillment

Finding harmony between nutrition, exercise, work, relationships, and personal fulfillment is key to living a balanced and fulfilling life. Here are some tips to help you achieve this harmony:

1. Prioritize self-care: Make self-care a priority in your daily routine. This includes taking time for yourself to relax, recharge, and engage in activities that bring you joy and fulfillment. Self-care can be as simple as reading a book, practicing mindfulness, or pursuing a hobby.
2. Plan and prioritize: Take a proactive approach to managing your time and commitments. Plan your schedule in advance and prioritize your tasks based on importance and urgency. This will help you allocate time for nutrition, exercise, work, relationships, and personal fulfillment.
3. Set realistic goals: Set goals that are attainable and aligned with your values and priorities. Break them down into smaller, actionable steps that you can work on consistently. This will help you stay focused and motivated while maintaining a sense of balance in your life.
4. Practice mindful eating: When it comes to nutrition, focus on mindful eating. Pay attention to your body's hunger and fullness cues, choose nourishing and satisfying foods, and eat with intention and awareness. Avoid using food as a coping mechanism or as a way to

deal with stress or emotions.

5. Incorporate physical activity into your routine: Find ways to incorporate physical activity into your daily routine, even if it's in small increments. This can include taking short walks during your breaks, using the stairs instead of the elevator, or engaging in active hobbies or sports. Exercise not only benefits your physical health but also contributes to your mental and emotional well-being.

6. Nurture relationships: Invest time and effort into building and nurturing relationships with your loved ones. Make quality time for your family and friends, listen actively, and communicate openly. Strong and supportive relationships can provide a sense of connection and fulfillment in your life.

7. Set boundaries: Establish healthy boundaries to protect your time, energy, and well-being. Learn to say no when necessary and prioritize your own needs and commitments. This will help prevent burnout and allow you to maintain balance in all aspects of your life.

8. Continuously reassess and adjust: Regularly reassess your priorities and commitments. Evaluate what is serving you and what may need adjustment. Be open to making changes and adapting your routines as needed to find the optimal balance that works for you.

Remember, finding harmony is an ongoing process, and it may require some trial and error. Be patient with yourself and give yourself permission to make adjustments along the way. By prioritizing self-care, setting realistic goals, and practicing mindful choices, you can find the harmony you seek and lead a fulfilling life that encompasses nutrition, exercise, work, relationships, and personal fulfillment.

The importance of stress reduction, relaxation, and self-care activities

In today's fast-paced world, stress reduction, relaxation, and self-care activities play a crucial role in maintaining our overall well-being. Here are some reasons why they are important:

1. Mental and emotional well-being: Stress can have a significant impact on our mental and emotional health. Engaging in stress reduction techniques, such as relaxation exercises, meditation, or engaging in hobbies, can help promote a sense of calm and inner peace. Taking time for self-care activities can also help alleviate symptoms of anxiety and depression, improve mood, and increase overall emotional well-being.

2. Physical health benefits: Chronic stress can have detrimental effects on our physical health. It can contribute to conditions such as high blood pressure, heart disease, and weakened immune system. Engaging in relaxation activities and self-care practices can help reduce stress hormones, lower blood pressure, and boost the immune system. It can also improve sleep quality, which is essential for overall health and well-being.

3. Improved productivity and focus: When we are constantly stressed and overwhelmed, our ability to concentrate and perform tasks efficiently can be compromised. Taking time for relaxation and self-care activities can help clear the mind, improve focus, and enhance productivity. It allows us to recharge our energy levels and approach our tasks with a renewed

sense of clarity and purpose.

4. Enhanced self-awareness and self-reflection: Engaging in self-care activities provides an opportunity for self-reflection and self-awareness. Taking time for ourselves allows us to tune into our needs, desires, and emotions. It helps us better understand ourselves, identify areas of improvement, and make necessary adjustments in our lives. Self-reflection promotes personal growth and helps us align our actions and priorities with our values and goals.

5. Stress management and resilience: Regular practice of stress reduction techniques and self-care activities can help build resilience and improve our ability to cope with challenging situations. It equips us with the tools and strategies needed to manage stress effectively, reduce its negative impact on our lives, and bounce back from setbacks more quickly.

6. Improved relationships: When we take care of ourselves and prioritize self-care, we are better equipped to engage in meaningful and fulfilling relationships. By reducing stress and enhancing our well-being, we can approach our interactions with others with a calmer and more positive mindset. This, in turn, can lead to improved communication, deeper connections, and more satisfying relationships.

7. Overall life satisfaction: Engaging in stress reduction, relaxation, and self-care activities contributes to our overall life satisfaction. It allows us to find balance in our lives, prioritize our well-being, and nurture ourselves. When we take the time to care for ourselves, we can experience greater joy, fulfillment, and a sense of purpose in our lives.

In summary, stress reduction, relaxation, and self-care activities are vital for our overall well-being. They support our mental, emotional, and physical health, enhance our relationships, and contribute to our overall life satisfaction. By making self-care a priority, we can lead more balanced, fulfilling lives and navigate the challenges of daily life with greater resilience and ease.

Developing a holistic approach to overall well-being

Developing a holistic approach to overall well-being involves taking a comprehensive and interconnected approach to address the different aspects of your physical, mental, and emotional health. Here are some key elements to consider in cultivating a holistic approach to well-being:

1. Physical health: Take care of your body by engaging in regular exercise, maintaining a balanced and nutritious diet, getting enough sleep, and attending to your medical and physical needs. This includes regular check-ups, staying hydrated, and managing any existing health conditions.

2. Mental and emotional health: Pay attention to your mental and emotional well-being by practicing stress management techniques, seeking support from trusted individuals or professionals when needed, and engaging in activities that promote mental clarity and emotional balance, such as meditation or journaling.

3. Social connections: Nurture your relationships and build a strong support network of friends, family, and community. Cultivate meaningful connections, engage in positive social interactions, and prioritize quality time with loved ones.

4. Intellectual stimulation: Continuously challenge your mind and stimulate your intellect by engaging in activities that expand your knowledge and skills. This could include reading, taking up a new hobby, learning a

musical instrument, or pursuing further education.

5. Spiritual well-being: Explore your values, beliefs, and sense of purpose. Engage in activities that promote spiritual growth and connection, such as meditation, mindfulness, or spending time in nature.

6. Work-life balance: Strive for a healthy balance between work, personal life, and leisure activities. Take regular breaks, set boundaries, and ensure that you allocate time for self-care and activities that bring you joy and fulfillment.

7. Environmental awareness: Foster an awareness of your impact on the environment and make choices that promote sustainability and a healthy planet. This includes reducing waste, conserving resources, and connecting with nature.

8. Self-care practices: Prioritize self-care activities that nourish your mind, body, and soul. This can include practices such as self-reflection, relaxation techniques, engaging in hobbies, spending time in nature, or pampering yourself with activities like taking a bath or getting a massage.

Remember, a holistic approach to well-being is about finding balance and integration across different areas of your life. It's about recognizing the interconnectedness of your physical, mental, and emotional health and taking proactive steps to nurture each aspect. By adopting a holistic perspective, you can enhance your overall well-being and lead a more fulfilling and purposeful life.

Final reflections on the journey to finding balance

Finding balance in life is an ongoing journey that requires self-awareness, intentionality, and adaptability. It's important to recognize that balance is not a fixed state, but rather a dynamic equilibrium that fluctuates over time. Here are some final reflections on the journey to finding balance:

1. Embrace flexibility: Balance is not about rigidly dividing your time and energy equally between all areas of your life. It's about being flexible and responsive to the changing demands and priorities that arise. Allow yourself to adjust and adapt as needed, and be open to reevaluating what balance means to you in different seasons of life.

2. Prioritize self-care: Self-care is not selfish; it's essential for maintaining balance and well-being. Make self-care a non-negotiable part of your routine, and prioritize activities that nourish your mind, body, and spirit. Remember that taking care of yourself is not only beneficial for you but also enables you to show up fully for others.

3. Set boundaries: Boundaries are crucial for protecting your time, energy, and mental well-being. Learn to say no to commitments that don't align with your priorities and values. Establish clear boundaries in your personal and professional life, and communicate them assertively and respectfully.

4. Cultivate mindfulness: Practice being present and fully

engaged in each moment. Mindfulness allows you to tune into your thoughts, emotions, and physical sensations, helping you make conscious choices and avoid becoming overwhelmed by distractions or external pressures. Cultivate mindfulness through meditation, deep breathing exercises, or simply paying attention to the present moment.

5. Seek support: You don't have to navigate the journey to balance alone. Seek support from trusted friends, family members, or professionals who can offer guidance, accountability, and perspective. Surround yourself with a supportive network that understands and respects your goals and values.

6. Embrace imperfection: Striving for balance doesn't mean achieving perfection in all areas of life. Accept that there will be times when things feel out of balance, and that's okay. Embrace the idea of "good enough" and give yourself permission to prioritize and make choices that align with your current needs and circumstances.

7. Reflect and adjust: Regularly take time to reflect on your current state of balance and evaluate what's working and what needs adjustment. Be willing to make changes and course-correct along the way. Remember that finding balance is a continuous process of learning, growth, and self-discovery.

Finding balance is a personal and individualized journey. It requires self-compassion, patience, and a willingness to experiment and learn from both successes and setbacks. By prioritizing self-care, setting boundaries, staying mindful, seeking support, and embracing imperfection, you can cultivate a sense of balance that allows you to live a fulfilling and meaningful life.

Encouragement to continue embracing a healthy lifestyle

Congratulations on taking the steps towards embracing a healthy lifestyle! It's not always an easy journey, but the rewards are truly worth it. As you continue on this path, here is some encouragement to help you stay motivated and committed:

1. Celebrate your progress: Take the time to acknowledge and celebrate the milestones you've reached along your journey. Whether it's losing a few pounds, running a faster mile, or making healthier food choices, each small step forward is a reason to be proud.

2. Focus on the process, not just the outcome: While reaching your goals is important, remember to find joy in the process itself. Embrace the daily habits, routines, and choices that contribute to your overall well-being. By enjoying the journey, you'll create a sustainable and fulfilling lifestyle.

3. Surround yourself with positivity: Surround yourself with people who support and encourage your healthy lifestyle. Seek out communities, online forums, or local groups that share your interests and goals. Having a support system can provide accountability, motivation, and inspiration.

4. Find activities you love: Exercise and physical activity shouldn't feel like a chore. Explore different activities until you find ones that you genuinely enjoy. Whether it's dancing, hiking, swimming, or playing a sport, find something that brings you joy and makes you excited to

move your body.

5. Practice self-compassion: Remember that progress is not always linear, and there will be ups and downs along the way. Be kind to yourself during challenging times or setbacks. Treat yourself with compassion, and focus on making sustainable changes rather than striving for perfection.

6. Embrace a growth mindset: Adopt a mindset that views challenges as opportunities for growth and learning. Embrace the idea that setbacks or obstacles are simply part of the journey. Approach each challenge with curiosity, and use it as a chance to discover new strategies and strengths.

7. Take care of your mental well-being: A healthy lifestyle is not just about physical health but also about nurturing your mental and emotional well-being. Make time for activities that bring you joy and relaxation, such as practicing mindfulness, journaling, spending time in nature, or connecting with loved ones.

Remember, a healthy lifestyle is a lifelong journey, and it's about finding balance, nourishing your body and mind, and enjoying the process. Stay committed, stay motivated, and know that you are capable of achieving and maintaining a healthy and fulfilling life.

Resources for ongoing support and further exploration

As you continue your journey towards a healthy lifestyle, there are many resources available to provide ongoing support and further exploration. Here are some resources that can help you:

1. Books: There are countless books on nutrition, fitness, mindset, and overall well-being. Look for reputable authors and titles that align with your interests and goals. Some popular books include "Atomic Habits" by James Clear, "Intuitive Eating" by Evelyn Tribole and Elyse Resch, and "The Four Agreements" by Don Miguel Ruiz.

2. Online Communities and Forums: Joining online communities and forums can provide a great platform for connecting with like-minded individuals, sharing experiences, and getting support and advice. Websites like Reddit, Healthline, and MyFitnessPal have active communities where you can ask questions, share successes, and learn from others.

3. Professional Support: Consider seeking guidance from professionals such as registered dietitians, personal trainers, therapists, or life coaches. These professionals can provide personalized advice, support, and expertise to help you navigate your specific goals and challenges.

4. Apps and Technology: There are numerous apps and digital tools available to track your progress, provide workout routines, offer healthy recipes, and even offer meditation and stress reduction techniques. Some

popular apps include MyFitnessPal, Headspace, and Nike Training Club.

5. Podcasts: Podcasts are a great way to learn, get inspired, and stay motivated on your health and wellness journey. There are many podcasts dedicated to nutrition, fitness, mindset, and personal growth. Some notable podcasts include "The Nutrition Diva's Quick and Dirty Tips for Eating Well and Feeling Fabulous," "The Model Health Show," and "The Tony Robbins Podcast."

6. Local Resources: Explore local resources in your community such as wellness centers, fitness classes, nutrition workshops, and support groups. Check out your local community center, gym, or health food store for information on events, classes, and resources.

Remember, everyone's journey is unique, so find the resources that resonate with you and support your specific goals and interests. Stay curious, keep learning, and be open to new ideas and approaches. With the right support and resources, you can continue to thrive and cultivate a healthy and fulfilling lifestyle.